MARCO ANTONIO QUIROZ AGUILAR
FERNADO AXIEL RODRÍGUEZ FILIO
JORGE FERNANDO MENDEZ GALVÁN

Impact on nutritional status from childhood to adolescence.

MARCO ANTONIO QUIROZ AGUILAR
FERNADO AXIEL RODRÍGUEZ FILIO
JORGE FERNANDO MENDEZ GALVÁN

Impact on nutritional status from childhood to adolescence.

Association between nutritional status in preschoolers and adolescents in rural localities of the State of Mexico.

ScienciaScripts

Cover image: www.ingimage.com

This book is a translation from the original published under ISBN 978-620-0-01590-7.

Publisher:
Sciencia Scripts
is a trademark of
Dodo Books Indian Ocean Ltd. and OmniScriptum S.R.L publishing group

120 High Road, East Finchley, London, N2 9ED, United Kingdom
Str. Armeneasca 28/1, office 1, Chisinau MD-2012, Republic of Moldova, Europe
Managing Directors: Ieva Konstantinova, Victoria Ursu
info@omniscriptum.com

Printed at: see last page
ISBN: 978-620-8-55451-4

ASSOCIATION BETWEEN NUTRITIONAL STATUS IN PRESCHOOLERS AND ADOLESCENTS IN RURAL LOCALITIES IN THE STATE OF MEXICO, 2002 - 2022.

AUTHORS:
DR. QUIROZ AGUILAR MARCO ANTONIO DR. RODRÍGUEZ FILIO FERNANDO AXIEL DR. MENDEZ GALVÁN JORGE FERNANDO

MEXICO CITY 28 NOVEMBER 2024

ACKNOWLEDGEMENTS

To Antúnez Reza María de los Ángeles, Moreno Beltrán Luz Angélica, Flores Salvador Monserrat, Sandoval Cerón Mariana, Moyao Morales Elideth, Alonso Delinea Yuridia, Bello Juárez Karen Adylene, Salgado Juárez Edwin Jair, P. Lic. Juárez Cervantes Erick Jaziel, students of the Centro Regional de Estudios Superiores Zona Norte (CRES ZN) of the Universidad Autónoma de Guerrero (UAGro) who showed great commitment in the collection of information for this thesis; in addition to the Escuela Superior de Acapulco (UAGro) to Lic. N. C. A. Ramírez Torres María Monserrat. To the

M. en C. S. De Sales Millán Amapola from the Autonomous Metropolitan University (UAM), Lic. De Sales Millán Carlos Antonio from UNITEC, Herrera Rodríguez Daniela Aylin, Trillo Salinas Mónica Yamileth and Morales Gómez José Agustín from UNITEC- MARINA. To the LN esp. Ped. Buendía Alemán Nidia Alejandra from the Universidad del Valle de México (UVM). To Trinidad Gil Adriana, Gil Santiago Rosa and Trinidad Gil María Concepción from the Consejo Nacional de Fomento Educativo (CONAFE) and to L.S.I. Sánchez Cayetano Luz María from Intercultural del Estado de México.

Without all of them this work would not have been possible, for which we are infinitely grateful, happy and hope that we have added a grain of sand to their life and academic experiences. Rest assured that their work has paid off.

Of course to our families, friends and close friends who encouraged us to continue in this process.

With love, Marco and Axiel.

SUMMARY

Due to the high prevalence of overweight and obesity at adolescent age in our country, different studies have been conducted from the perspective of risk factors (type of locality of residence, welfare conditions, family history of obesity, physical activity, screen time). This study aims to evaluate the nutritional status and socioeconomic conditions at adolescent age and compare it with the nutritional status of preschool children in rural localities of the State of Mexico. A retrospective cross-sectional observational study was carried out, including 515 children from 27 localities distributed in three municipalities of the State of Mexico from a sample universe of 1740 preschoolers, of whom at least two anthropometric data on weight and height measured between 2002 and 2009 were available. For the final measurements, we worked with adolescents between 12 and 16 years of age, with parents or guardians present, and obtained the following data: identification, housing characteristics, family food resources, parents' general data, postnatal information on the adolescent and anthropometric data. The most relevant results found were that during the first years of age, 47.8% of the children had <2 D.E. in malnutrition with the height-for-age indicator, while 20.2% are undernourished with the height-for-age indicator.overweight or obese according to BMI/E, in adolescents 21.2% have low height (<2 D.E.); according to BMI/E 27.2% are overweight plus obesity, with respect to the lower extremities 17.9% are brachyskeletal and 30.9% have a waist-to-height ratio in the risk category, the average number of children born alive in the families interviewed is 5; 12.9% of the adolescents had low birth weight and the average number of children born alive in the families interviewed is 5; 12.9% of the adolescents had low birth weight and the average number of children born alive in the families interviewed is 5; 12.9% of the adolescents had low birth weight and the average number of children born alive in the families interviewed is 5; 12.9% of the adolescents had low birth weight. weekly family income is 894.00 pesos. There is a significant relationship $P<0.05$ when comparing heights at both ages. Although childhood nutritional status has a stronger association with possible effects on adolescent height than BMI/E, short stature and short limbs are associated with overweight and obesity at adolescent age, while acceptable waist size index decreases the likelihood of being overweight and obese. It is necessary to study the current diet of adolescents in order to know the effect it has on their nutritional status, as well as pre-post natal and socio-economic data at preschool age. Nutritional surveillance needs to have the capacity to collect more specific information that allows for a better understanding of the conditions in which children develop and the possibility of intervening positively in the health and poverty cycle. It is vitally important to create public policies that guarantee maternal and perinatal health, family planning, and improve the income of families in rural communities in order to reduce low height in pre-school age, overweight and obesity in adolescence and chronic non-degenerative diseases in adulthood.

INDEX

CHAPTER 1

CONSTRUCTION OF THE PROBLEM

1.1 Background

In 1990 David Barker linked intrauterine growth retardation, low birth weight and preterm birth to high blood pressure, coronary heart disease and non-insulin dependent diabetes in middle age. The growth and development of the foetus is determined by three factors: the nutritional status of the pregnant woman, placental function and the ability of the foetus to utilise nutrients. An in utero insult could lead to abnormal programming of systems and be expressed in the life of the individual (Moreno-Villares & Dalmau, 2001).Studies have shown that dysregulation in the availability of energy substrates, both in prenatal and postnatal life, predispose to the development of metabolic and hormonal adaptation processes that persist throughout life and are related to the development of chronic degenerative diseases. Obesity has been related to morbid processes that are established from an adverse intrauterine environment, either by placental insufficiency that causes the development of adaptive processes that often persist throughout postnatal life (Garibay-Nieto & Miranda-Lora, 2008).Individuals who have developed intrauterine growth retardation (IUGR) tend to have a lower body mass index (BMI) than those who hada higher birth weight, however, they tend to present an accumulation of predominantly central and visceral adipose tissue, with a very significant decrease in muscle mass that becomes evident from puberty onwards (Garibay-Nieto & Miranda-Lora, 2008).A study in an urban area of Brazil showed that height at birth, height attained in infancy and particularly rapid growth velocity from birth to 20 months of age are associated with increased prevalence of overweight and obesity in adolescence (Monteiro et al., 2003).A study in a rural population in the State of Oaxaca shows significant secular increases in the height, sitting height and estimated leg length of children and adolescents between 1978 and 2000, and although it is not specified which changes contributed to the growth, it suggests that improvements in health, nutrition and living conditions over 20 years are the contributing causes of these secular gains in growth (Malina R. M. et al., 2004).It has been observed that the influence of maternal weight determines the ratio of birth weight in the newborn and subsequent BMI, which is related to the increased energy intake of energy substrates in the couple. Prenatal risk factors, such as age, parity, incidence of pre-eclampsia, smoking, socio-economic status and obesity, are all determinants of alterations in BMI. metabolism and glucose tolerance and obesity in their offspring (Garibay-Nieto & Miranda-Lora, 2008a).Breastfeeding is known to be a protective factor for the incidence of obesity in infants, these children show a lower weight gain and body fat, it is suggested that it could protect against childhood obesity and its associated comorbidities in adulthood (Garibay-Nieto & Miranda-Lora, 2008), (Labraña et al., 2020).In addition, there is a two-way causal relationship between poverty and ill-health - poverty causes ill-health and ill-health sustains poverty. Individuals or families with low incomes, with little or no access, availability or poor quality of health services, will have poor health and unhealthy dietary practices, leading to poor health, nutrition and multiparity outcomes, resulting in low wages, increased vulnerability to disease, higher health care costs and thus continuing the cycle of health and poverty (Wagstaff, 2002).So it is known that child growth is not always linear, and when there is a deficit in it, in order to demonstrate its restoration, 4 criteria would have to be met: first, to know the condition that inhibited growth, second, to know the speed at which it was reduced, third, to have a stage of relief or composition of the inhibition condition and finally, that there is a higher than normal growth rate in a subsequent period (Frongillo et al., 2019).

1.2 Approach of the Problem.

Chronic undernutrition in preschoolers continues to be a public health problem in Mexico; the decline that had been occurring was interrupted by data from the National Health and Nutrition Survey 2018-19 (ENSANUT 2018-19). The national prevalence in 2012 13.6% and 2018-19 it was 14.2% (Cuevas- Nasu et al., 2021). In rural communities in Mexico, 17.5% of children under five years of age are stunted (Shamah, 2018). The factors associated with short stature in children under five years of age were studied by dividing the population into children under 24 months and 24-59 months, and the factors were grouped into three blocks: household and geographic, maternal and individual. With respect to geographical factors, the prevalences observed in rural areas for children under 24 months were among the highest (18.0%), and in the southern region of the country (18.7%) for each of the age groups; these are highly marginalised localities and belong to the lowest economic tercile. According to maternal factors, the prevalence was higher in children of indigenous mothers 30.2% and 27.3% for each age group respectively, and they are also mothers with low levels of schooling. And in individual factors, 30.3% of children 24 months do not have a diverse diet and are chronically malnourished; there is also moderate and severe food insecurity. 22.9% have low height when they are anaemic (Cuevas-Nasu et al., 2021). The presence of overweight and obesity in adolescents reaches 38.4%. In rural areas, the reported prevalence of overweight women is 24.4% and obesity is 24.4%. 14.0%, for males a prevalence of overweight of 17.6% and obesity of 13.2% was observed (Shamah, 2018). Risk factors associated with overweight and obesity in adolescents between 12 and 19 years of age have been studied, overweight and obesity in the mother, increased screen time, average well-being index (housing characteristics, possession of goods and services in the home), as well as when the percentage of energy consumed comes from free sugars and increased protein intake, were associated with overweight and obesity in adolescence. The fact that it is a cross-sectional study does not allow causality to be inferred (Shamah & Rivera, 2020).Chávez denounced that there are those who support the hypothesis that a child who suffered moderate

malnutrition at an early age will only lose height, and in adulthood will have a "scar" that will make him/her <small but healthy>, will become balanced, will require less food, they affirm that his/her mental and social underdevelopment is more of a cultural than functional nature and that he/she will be able to become a good agricultural worker (Chávez & Muñoz, 2007). Contrary to this hypothesis, it is known that child undernutrition affects survival, is associated with different functional deficiencies, such as muscular, skeletal and immunological development, and affects their cognitive and intellectual capacities (Chávez & Muñoz, 2007), (UNICEF, 2019).
Child malnutrition forces the affected child to seek physiological stability (homeorresis) as a defence measure, sacrificing height to continue developing, compared to children of the same age and ethnic group who have not presented such a condition; this balance does not allow the organic and functional characteristicsare normal (Chávez & Muñoz, 2007), (Cravioto, 2003). In rural communities, the study "Effect of malnutrition on children's neurointegrative development" positively associates the mother's low level of education with her child's short stature (Cravioto, 2003).With regard to changes in body dimensions it is known that there is a higher ratio of upper to lower body segment, as growth cartilage requires a lot of energy, lack of energy affects the growth of long bones, this difference remains throughout life so in theory it could be measured at any stage of life, but there are no reference standards. Decreased growth hormone secretion is also diminished in severe malnutrition, which adds to the deficiency in physical growth (Chavez & Munoz, 2007).There are two perspectives on the critical windows for nutritional interventions to prevent stunting, on the one hand (Prentice et al., 2013) mention that there is an extended pubertal growth phase, i.e. height can make a substantial recovery between 24 months and middle childhood even in the absence of nutritional interventions, on the other hand (Leroy et al., 2013) refute by commenting that there is no evidence to suggest that this happens after 24 months of age in stunted populations in low- and middle-income countries. Rapid weight gain in the neonatal and infancy stage is a risk factor for increased adiposity and obesity in childhood and adulthood. In preterm patients, early postnatal growth (first three months of life), and to a lesser extent late postnatal growth, was found to be associated with higher body fat percentage, abdominal fat and BMI at 19 years of age. In a cohort study, the period between birth and the first week of life was found to be potentially critical for the development of obesity, finding that weight gain at this stage is strongly associated with overweight in adulthood (Garibay-Nieto & Miranda-Lora, 2008). Restoring growth, in addition to eliminating the inhibiting condition(s) and the higher than normal gain in growth velocity, involves improving the conditions under which children grow, develop at school and adolescent age (Frongillo et al., 2019).Rapid growth leads to a "catch-up dilemma", which may be beneficial in the short term by reducing child morbidity and mortality, but risky in the long term because of the presence of chronic non-communicable diseases in adulthood (Monteiro et al., 2003).

1.2.1 research question

Is there a relationship between the nutritional status of adolescents and their nutritional status at preschool age?

1.3 Justification

Anthropometric assessment measures the overall dimensions and composition of the human body, variables that are affected by nutrition throughout the life cycle. Anthropometric indicators measure child and adolescent physical growth by total body mass and body composition in both health and disease (Ravasco et al., 2010). Due to the high prevalence of overweight and obesity at adolescent age in our country, we consider it important to evaluate the predisposition to this public health problem with respect to nutritional status at preschool age. Studies have been conducted on this topic from the perspective of risk factors (type of locality of residence, welfare conditions, family history of obesity, physical activity, screen time), with this study we aim to address the association of nutritional status in early childhood and the effect it has on adolescence.

1.4 Objectives

1.4.1 Objective general

To assess the nutritional status and socioeconomic conditions at adolescent age and compare it with the nutritional status at preschool age in the population of rural localities in the State of Mexico.

1.4.2 Objectives specific

Measure and classify nutritional status in early childhood and adolescence Compare nutritional status in early childhood vs. nutritional status in adolescence.Assess variables associated with nutritional status.

1.5 Hypothesis

There is an association between childhood and adolescent nutritional status.

CHAPTER 2

METHODOLOGY

2.1 Material and methods

2.1.1 Type of study

Retrospective cross-sectional observational study.

2.1.2 Description of the cohort

Children from 27 localities distributed in three municipalities (San José del Rincón, San Felipe del Progreso and Villa Victoria) were included. The study universe consisted of 1740 children, for whom we had at least two anthropometric data on weight and height measured between 2002 and 2009, i.e. when they were between 0 and 5 years of age.For the final measurements, we worked with a sample of 535 adolescents aged between 12 and 16 years at the time, representing 30.7% of the study universe, who were surveyed and the following data were obtained: identification, housing characteristics, family food resources, parents' general data, postnatal information on the adolescent and anthropometric data.

2.1.3 Collection of the information

The fieldwork for the survey and anthropometry was carried out by students and staff of the nutrition degree of the University.Autónoma de Guerrero, Universidad Tecnológica and Universidad del Valle de Toluca, who were previously trained and standardised. In order to obtain data in the survey, home visits were made to mothers, fathers or any adult who knew all the information regarding the economic and nutritional conditions of the adolescent.

2.1.4 Variables of study

The study variables were collected through the survey at the time of the visit (Annex 1). A letter of consent (Appendix 2) and a letter of agreement (Appendix 3) were requested to be signed. If the adolescent not at home at the time of the visit, the measurements were taken at a later date.

2.1.4.1 Modules of the survey

The aspects considered in order to obtain the information and fulfil the objectives of this research made up the different modules and variables of the survey, which are listed below:

1. Identification data: Municipality, locality, identification number and date of visit.

2. Identification of the adolescent: Name of the interviewee, name of the adolescent, CURP, date of birth and sex.

3. Characteristics of the dwelling: materials used in construction, number of rooms, separation of kitchen, ventilation, presence of animals, energy. electricity, source of heat for cooking, source of water supply, excreta disposal, rubbish disposal, home ownership and property ownership.
4. Household food resources: Weekly food expenditure, participation in food assistance programmes, raising food animals, growing food at home.
5. General data on the adolescent's parents: Age, number of children, marital status, language, social security, schooling of mother, father and adolescent.
6. Adolescent postnatal information: Gestation, birth weight, breastfeeding and complementary feeding.

2.1.4.2. Anthropometry

The following anthropometric measures were considered: weight, height, sitting height and waist circumference of fathers, mothers and adolescents. Weight: The amount of matter in the body. It is calculated by measuring the weight, i.e. the force exerted by matter in a standard gravitational field. The measurement shall be taken without shoes and with as little clothing as possible. The subject shall stand in the centre of the scale and remain stationary during the measurement. The measurement is recorded when the numbers on the digital scale stabilise. SECA model 872 scales were used, with a maximum capacity of 200 kilograms and an accuracy of 0.05 grams.Size: This is the perpendicular distance between the transverse planes of the vertex point and the bottom of the feet. The person shall be shoeless and shall stand with heels together, legs straight and shoulders relaxed. The back of the subject (heels, shoulder blades and head) shall be close to the vertical surface of the stadiometer. The head should be positioned in the horizontal Frankfort plane, which is presented by a line between the lowest point of the eye socket and the tragus. The subject is instructed to take a deep breath in and out and, while holding the head in the Frankfort plane, the anthropometrist applies moderate traction on the mastoid process upwards. Head ornaments should be removed. SECA model 213 stadiometers with a maximum capacity of 2015 centimetres and an accuracy of 1 millimetre were used.Seated height: This is the perpendicular distance between the transverse planes of the vertex point and the lower region of the buttocks, with the subject seated. The subject is instructed to take a deep breath in and out and, while holding the head in the Frankfort plane, the anthropometrist applies a moderate upward traction on the mastoid process. Care should be taken to ensure that the subject does not contract the buttocks or apply pressure with the legs. The stadiometer square is placed on the vertex, compressing the hair. SECA model 213 stadiometers with a maximum capacity of 2015 centimetres and an accuracy of 1 millimetre were used.Waist circumference: The circumference of the abdomen at its narrowest point, between the lower lateral costal margin and the top of the iliac crest, perpendicular to the longitudinal axis of the trunk. The measurement is taken at the midpoint between the lower lateral costal margin and the iliac crest. The subject should breathe normally and the measurement is taken at the end of a normal exhalation and with the abdominal musculature relaxed. SECA model 201 measuring tapes were used, with a maximum capacity of 205 centimetres and an accuracy of 1 millimetre.

2.1.5 Criteria for inclusion

- Who had their nutritional status assessed between 2002 and 2009.

- Who live in the selected localities of the municipalities of Villa Victoria, San José del Rincón and San Felipe del Progreso, State of Mexico.
- Have at least two anthropometric height in their pre-school years.

2.1.6 exclusion criteria

□Adolescent not present to take anthropometric measurements

□Not being the right informant for the interview.

□Children with pathologies that do not allow anthropometric measurements.

2.1.8 Plan for analysis

Cut-off points and classification of nutritional status of preschoolers and adolescents. According to the WHO reference population, weight-for-age (W/F) and height-for-age (H/F) Z-scores were calculated for preschoolers under five years of age based on anthropometric measurements. In adolescents, body mass index for age (BMI/A) Z-scores were calculated. The cut-off points used to compare nutritional status were as follows:

P/E Z-score P/E Point of State of Cut nutrition		T/E Z-score T/E Point of State of Cut nutrition		BMI/E Z-score BMI/E Point of State of Cut nutrition	
-3 a -5	Severe or severe	-2 a -5	Baja	-2 a -5	Severe thinness
-2 a - 2.99 -1 a - 1.99 -0.99 a 0.99	Moderate Mild Normal	-0.99 a - 1.99 -0.99 a .99 1 a 1.99	Slightly low Normal Slightly high	-0.99 a - 1.99 -0.99 a .99 1 a 1.99	Thinness Normal weight Overweight
1 a 1.99	Overweight	2 a 5	High	2 a 5	Obesity
2 a 5	Obesity				

Cut-off points and sitting size classification

With respect to sitting height, the skeletal or Manouvrier index was used, which relates the length of the trunk to the length of the lower limb, measured as the difference between height and sitting height. The division of individuals according to their skeletal index is as follows:

Cut-off point Ranking

< 84.9 Brachyskeletal

85 - 89.9 Mesoskeletal

> 90 Macroskeletal

Cut-off points and classification of waist size index.

The cut-off point of > 0.5 classifies them as elevated and correlates with increased adverse cardiovascular and metabolic risk factors, independent of age, gender and ethnicity. (Curilem, 2016).
Cut-off points and socio-economic status classification

The socio-economic level model provides an overview of the level of well-being of households in the country, both in the rural and urban strata. It is constructed from 6 variables:

• Educational level of the head of household

• Number of complete bathrooms in the dwelling

• Number of cars in the household (understood as the sum of cars, vans and pick-up trucks in the household)

• Internet connection in the household

• Number of working household members over 14 years of age

• Number of bedrooms in the dwelling

According to the respondent's answers in these variables, corresponding points are assigned to each response option, which are then added up. This sum will be contrasted with the following cut-off points to assign the respective household to its corresponding socio-economic level:

Socio-economic status Cut-off points for classification

Socio-economic status	Cut-off points for classification
Marginal	0 a 47
Lower bass	48 a 94
Upper bass	95 a 115
Medium	116 a 140
Low medium	141 a 167
Medium high	168 a 201
High	202 or more

The statistical analysis was carried out with the SPSS (Statistical Package for the Social Sciences) version 20 package.

CHAPTER 3

RESULTS

3.1 Results

From a universe of 1740 adolescents, a sub-sample of 515 subjects was taken from27 localities distributed in three municipalities of the State of Mexico by marginalisation index, reaching a coverage of 29.6% (see table 1).

Table 1. Distribution of coverage, universe and study sample by marginalisation index, locality and municipality.locality

MunicipalityName of the	Marginalisation index	Universe	Sample	% coverage
Calvario Del				
Carmen Bo. El		208	61	29.3
Picacho				
St. JeromeUpper Bonchete		147	44	29.9
San Juan Cote Centre		34	10	29.4
Dotegiare		56	19	33.9
Las Palomas		75	21	28.0
Rancheria El Medium		11	3	27.3
Rioyos Buenavista		37	13	35.1
San Juan Cote Ejido		42	15	35.7
Tlalchichilpa		59	18	30.5
Three Stars		48	11	22.9
Barrio Santa Ana Pueblo Nuevo		41	11	26.8
La Esperanza		44	20	45.5
San Miguel Water Blessed		56	11	19.6
The Forty-Four		21	5	23.8
Las Rosas Medium		134	40	29.9
Rancheria Las Rosas		42	10	23.8
San Felipe De Jesus		38	15	39.5
Puentecillas Neighbourhood		88	23	26.1
Loma De La Rosa		34	23	67.6

	San Luis El Alto	Medium	53	17	32.1
Total		1740		515	29.6

The following table shows the percentage distribution of socio-economic level by municipality in the State of Mexico, where it was found that the population is mainly concentrated in the two categories "marginal and low-inferior" with 72% of the surveyed families.

Table 2. Distribution of socio-economic status of adolescents by municipality in the State of Mexico.

Socio-economic level

	n	%	n	%	n	%	N	%
Marginal	51	22.4	46	38.0	59	35.5	156	30.3
Lower bass	120	52.6	62	51.2	84	50.6	266	51.7
Upper bass	28	12.3	4	3.3	12	7.2	44	8.5
Medium	6	2.6	1	0.8	3	1.8	10	1.9
Low medium	21	9.2	7	5.8	8	4.8	36	7.0
Medium high	1	0.4	1	0.8	0	0.0	2	0.4
High	1	0.4	0	0.0	0	0.0	1	0.2
Total	228	100.0	121	100.0	166	100.0	515	100.0

Source: Fieldwork

Table 3 shows the distribution of adolescents by age and sex, with the highest prevalence in the female population at 55.1%.

Table 3. Distribution of adolescents by age and sex.

Female Male Total Age in years completed

n		%	n	%	N
12	34	50.0	34	50.0	68
13	72	51.1	69	48.9	141
14	95	57.2	71	42.8	166
15	57	57.6	42	42.4	99
16	26	63.4	15	36.6	41
Total	284	55.1	231	44.9	515

Source: Fieldwork Regarding the characteristics of the construction materials of the dwellings in the Mazahua zone, the most prevalent are concrete slabs (76.3%), brick or block walls (86.6%) and cement or solid floor (88.9%) (Table 4).

Table 4. Characteristics of the construction materials used in the housing of higher prevalence.

Housing construction materials	N	n	%
Concrete slab or joists with vault (Roof)	515	393	76.3
Partition, brick, block, stone, quarry, cement or concrete (Walls)	515	446	86.6
Cement or firm (Floor)	515	458	88.9

Source: Fieldwork

Table 5 shows the percentage distribution of overcrowding in the surveyed dwellings in the Mazahua area, 31.2% were classified as having some type of overcrowding.

Table 5. Percentage distribution of the level of overcrowding in housing.

	N	%
No overcrowding	353	68.8
Low overcrowding	145	28.3
High overcrowding	15	2.9
Total	513	100.0

No overcrowding < 3 inhabitants per room. Low overcrowding 3 to 5 inhabitants per room. High overcrowding > 5 inhabitants per room.

Source: Fieldwork

Distribution of the characteristics of the dwelling, 81.6% of the surveyed families have a separate kitchen and 17.9% have animals inside the dwelling (Table 6).

Table 6. Percentage distribution of the characteristics of the dwelling.

Housing

	N	%
Ventilation	465	90.3
Animals inside	92	17.9
Electric power	495	96.1
Separate kitchen	420	81.6

Source: Fieldwork

According to the distribution of where the kitchen is located when it is separated from the dwelling, 56.9% have it on a roof (Table 7). **Table 7. Percentage distribution when there is a separate kitchen in dwelling.**

Separate kitchen

	N	%
Tejaban or techito	239	56.9
Corridor or corridor	69	16.4
Open air	33	7.9
No cooking in the dwelling	9	2.1
No reply	70	16.7
Total	420	100.0

Source: Fieldwork

Table 8 shows the distribution of fuel used for cooking in the household, 86.8% of households use firewood for cooking.

Table 8. Percentage distribution of fuel used for cooking in the household.

Cooking fuel

	N	%
Firewood	447	86.8
Cylinder or stationary gas	64	12.4
Natural or piped gas	3	0.6
Coal	1	0.2
Total	515	100.0

Source: Fieldwork

Table 9 shows the distribution of the type of cooker used for cooking in the dwelling, 73.4% of households prepare their food on an open fire with or without a chimney and hood.

Table 9. Percentage distribution of the type of cooker used for cooking in the dwelling.

Type of cooker

	N	%
Open fire or oven without chimney or hood	201	39.0
Open fire or oven with chimney or hood	177	34.4
Gas cooker or grill	125	24.3
Closed furnace with chimney	9	1.7
Electric cooker or grill	3	0.6
Total	515	100.0

Source: Fieldwork

Table 10 shows the distribution of piped water reaching the household, with 49.7% of the respondents having piped water reaching their land.

Table 10. Percentage distribution of piped water reaching the dwelling.

Piped water

	N	%
Only on the ground	256	49.7
No piped water	191	37.1
Inside the house	68	13.2
Total	515	100.0

Source: Fieldwork

Table 11 shows the origin of the water used in the household, 97.8% is obtained from a well or from the public water service.

Table 11. Percentage distribution of the origin of piped water reaching the dwelling.

Origin of where piped water comes from

	N	%
Well	224	69.1
Public water utility	93	28.7
Other housing	5	1.5
Pipe	1	0.3
Other place	1	0.3
Total	324	100.0

Source: Fieldwork Table 12 shows the distribution of where they carry the water they use.

In the household, 96.3% of the surveyed households draw their water from a well or from a public tap.

Table 12. Percentage distribution of where they carry the water they use in the home

The water they use in the house is carried by

	N	%
It is taken or carried from a well.	163	85.3
It is carried from a communal tap.	21	11.0
It is brought by a pipe	3	1.6
It is carried from a river, stream or lake.	2	1.0
It is brought from another dwelling	1	0.5
Catching the rain	1	0.5
Total	191	100.0

Source: Fieldwork

In table 13 we can observe the distribution of excreta disposal in the dwelling, 36.3% of the population practises fecalism at ground level.

Table 13. Percentage distribution of excreta disposal in the dwelling.

Excreta disposal

	N	%
Septic tank or septic tank (biodigester)	303	58.8
Faecalism at ground level	187	36.3
Drainage from the public network	17	3.3
Pipe leading to a gully or crevice	7	1.4
Pipeline leading to a river, lake or sea	1	0.2
Total	515	100.0

Source: Fieldwork

Table 14 shows the characteristics of the sanitary facilities in the dwelling, 59.6% of the toilets cannot be flushed.

Table 14. Percentage distribution of the characteristics of the sanitary service to the dwelling.

Characteristics of the health service

	N	%
No water can be poured	307	59.6
Water is poured in a bucket	163	31.7
It has a direct water discharge	45	8.7
Total	515	100.0

Source: Fieldwork

Table 15 shows the distribution of sharing the toilet, 90.7% of the respondents report that they do not share the toilet in the dwelling.

Table 15. Percentage distribution of sanitation service if shared with other dwellings.

Shared health service

	N	%
No	467	90.7
Yes	48	9.3
Total	515	100.0

Source: Fieldwork The following table shows how the rubbish is collected, 94.4% of Respondents report burning the rubbish or throwing it in the collection truck (Table 16).

Table 16. Percentage distribution of waste generated in the household.

Rubbish in the dwelling

	N	%
They burn it	348	67.6
It is collected by a rubbish truck or cart	138	26.8
It is dumped in a container or depot	13	2.5
They bury it	12	2.3
It is dumped in the public rubbish dump	1	0.2
They throw it into the ravine or crevasse.	1	0.2
It is thrown into the river, lake or dam.	1	0.2
It is dumped in a vacant lot or street.	1	0.2
Total	515	100.0

Source: Fieldwork

Table 17 shows the type of housing that the household has, 87.0% of the respondents say that they own their home.

Table 17. Percentage distribution of housing type.

Housing is?

	N	%
Own	448	87.0
Borrowed	49	9.5
Another situation	6	1.2
Intestate or in dispute	6	1.2
Own, but they are paying for it	4	0.8
Rented	2	0.4
Total	515	100.0

Source: Fieldwork

Table 18 shows the possessions owned by the household, 15.5% of the households own a car.

Table 18. Percentage distribution of possessions held by the household.

Possessions

	N	%
Automobile	80	15.5
Internet	63	12.2
Closed or cab-over van	17	3.3
Box van	26	5.0

Source: Fieldwork

Table 19 shows the averages of household income and food expenditure per week, as well as persons living in the dwelling, the average weekly household income is 894.1 pesos.

Table 19. Average income, expenditure and persons living in the .

Household economy and number of persons living in the dwelling	NAverage Minimum MaximumS.D.				
Income	513	894.1	100	3000	583.3
Expenditure	515	551.9	100	2000	297.5
Persons living in the dwelling	515	5.8	2	16	2.2

Source: Fieldwork

Table 20 shows the distribution of whether any member of the household receives any type of food aid, 93.2% of the households report not having any type of food aid.

Table 20. Percentage distribution if any member of the household receives food support.

Receives food aid

	N	%
No	480	93.2
Yes	35	6.8
Total	515	100.0

Source: Fieldwork

Table 21 shows the distribution of the programmes that the family currently receives. 68.6% of the families reported receiving food from DIF or an NGO.

Table 21. Percentage distribution of types of food assistance programmes received by a household member.

Programmes

	N	%
DIF food pantries	14	40.0
NGO food supplies	10	28.6
Hot school breakfasts	6	17.1
Cold school breakfasts	3	8.6
Welfare	2	5.7
Total	35	100.0

Source: Fieldwork

Table 22 shows the distribution of the programmes that the adolescent received during his or her lifetime, 100% of the adolescents surveyed received food parcels from DIF and 7.8% of adolescents report having received cold school breakfasts.

Table 22. Percentage distribution of the types of food assistance programmes received by the adolescent over the course of his or her lifetime.

Programmes

	N	%
DIF food pantries	515	100.0
Cold school breakfasts	40	7.8
Hot school breakfasts	26	5.0
Prospera	19	3.7
Opportunities	15	2.9
NGO food supplies	12	2.3
Community canteen	8	1.6
Progress	6	1.2
LICONSA milk	5	1.0
Benito Juarez	1	0.2

Source: Fieldwork

Table 23 shows the distribution of animal for family food, 75.1% of the surveyed families mentioned raising animals for family food.

Table 23. Percentage distribution of food animal husbandry.

Raising animals for food

	N	%
Yes	387	75.1
No	128	24.9
Total	515	100.0

Source: Fieldwork

Table 24 shows the distribution of the type of animal husbandry, 69.1% (small livestock) and 55.9% (large livestock) both are for family consumption. **Table 24. Percentage distribution of the type of animal husbandry for food.**

Small livestock

Large livestock

Animal husbandry

n		%	n	%
Self-consumption	253	69.1	19	55.9
Both	105	28.7	12	35.3
Sale	8	2.2	3	8.8
Total	366	100.0	34	100.0

Source: Fieldwork

Table 25 shows the distribution of food cultivation for food, 77.1% of the households do grow food for their diet.

Table 25. Percentage distribution if growing food for food

Food crops

	N	%
Yes	397	77.1
No	118	22.9
Total	515	100.0

Source: Fieldwork

Table 26 shows the distribution of the type of crops grown for food, 93.8% of families grow basic grains for their own consumption.

Table 26. Percentage distribution of the type of crops grown for food.

Fruit Vegetables Staple grains Food crops

n % n %					n	%
Self-consumption	37	94.9	53	85.5	335	93.8
Both	2	5.1	9	14.5	20	5.6
Sale	0	0.0	0	0.0	2	0.6
Total	39	100.0	62	100.0	357	100.0

Source: Fieldwork

The following table shows the average age of the parents of the adolescents, as well as of the adolescent himself, the average age of the mothers of the adolescents is 41 years and the average age of the fathers is 43 years (Table 27).

Table 27. Average age of mother, father and adolescent.

Age referred to in years completed	N	Average	Minimum	Maximum	D.E.
Mother's age	502	41	27	64	6.791
Father's age	431	43	29	65	7.185
Age of the adolescent	515	14	12	17	1.11

Source: Fieldwork

Table 28 shows the average number of live births, with an average of 5 children born per family.

Table 28. Average number of children born alive to the mother of the mother of the

adolescent.		
Number of live births	N	Average Minimum Maximum D.E.
Adolescent's mother	503	5 1 15 2.387

Source: Fieldwork

Table 29 shows the distribution of the marital status of the adolescents' parents, as well as the adolescents themselves: 92.3% of the parents are married or in union, while 99.0% of the adolescents are single.

Table 29. Percentage distribution of marital status of parents and adolescent.

Parents

Teenager

Marital status

	n	%	n	%
Married	279	55.6	3	0.6
Free union	184	36.7	2	0.4
Single	19	3.8	510	99.0
Widower	12	2.4	0	0.0
Divorced	8	1.6	0	0.0
Total	502	100.0	515	100.0

Source: Fieldwork

Table 30 presents the language distribution of the parents of the adolescents and the adolescent, the mothers of the adolescents have the highest prevalence (40.6%) of Spanish and Mazahua (bilingual), 60.3% of the parents speak Spanish and 91.1% of the adolescents speak Spanish.

Table 30. Percentage distribution of parents' and adolescent's language.

Mum Dad Adolescent Language

n%n%n%

English	296	58.8	260	60.3	469	91.1
Bilingual	204	40.6	171	39.7	46	8.9
Indigenous	3	0.6	0	0.0	0	0.0
Total	503	100.0	431	100.0	515	100.0

Source: Fieldwork Table 31 shows the distribution of social security of the parents of the children of the children who were born in the country.

adolescents, as well as the adolescents themselves, an average of 89.6% of the study subjects do not have social security.

Table 31. Percentage distribution of parents' social security and theadolescent. Security

Mum Dad Teenager

social	n	%	n	%	n	%
No Security	451	89.7	376	87.2	474	92.0
Don't Know	36	7.2	33	7.7	27	5.2
IMSS	10	2.0	13	3.0	8	1.6
Other Institution	5	1.0	8	1.9	5	1.0
ISSSTE	1	0.2	1	0.2	1	0.2
Total	503	100.0	431	100.0	515	100.0

Source: Fieldwork

Table 32 shows the distribution of parental and adolescent schooling: 34.4% vs. 33.8% of mothers vs. fathers have completed primary school and 47.6% of adolescents have incomplete secondary school at the time of the interview.

Table 32. Percentage distribution of parents' and adolescent's schooling.

Mum Dad Adolescent Schooling

N % n % n %

No education	66	13.1	39	9.1	1	0.2
Preschool	5	1.0	6	1.4	3	0.6
Primary complete	173	34.4	145	33.8	150	29.1
Primary incomplete	136	27.0	102	23.8	11	2.1
Secondary complete	106	21.1	108	25.2	80	15.5
Secondary incomplete	11	2.2	15	3.5	245	47.6
High School complete	5	1.0	8	1.9	2	0.4
High School incomplete	1	0.2	2	0.5	23	4.5
Bachelor's degree complete	0	0.0	4	0.9	0	0.0
Total	503	100.0	429	100.0	515	100.0

Source: Fieldwork

Table 33 shows the distribution of gestation time, 94.4% of the adolescents had a normal gestation time.

Table 33. Percentage distribution of gestation time during pregnancy.

Gestation

	N	%
Normal	486	94.4
Premature	27	5.2
Post-mature	2	0.4
Total	515	100.0

Source: Fieldwork Table 34 shows the distribution of adolescent birth weight, 87.1% of which was in the first year of life, and 87.1% in the second year of life. of adolescents had a normal birth weight.

Table 34. Percentage distribution of adolescent birth weight.

Birth weight

	N	%
Normal	445	87.1
Underweight	66	12.9
Total	511	100.0
		Source: Fieldwork

Table 35 shows the distribution of whether the adolescent was breastfed, 96.9% of adolescents were breastfed.

Percentage distribution if the adolescent was breastfed.

Maternal breast

	N	%
Yes	499	96.9
No	16	3.1
Total	515	100.0
		Source: Fieldwork

Table 36 presents the distribution of the type of breastfeeding the child received, 72.2% of the adolescents were breastfed and 3.1% were bottle-fed.

Table 36. Percentage distribution of the type of breastfeeding the child received

adolescent.							
	Chest		Mixed		Baby bottle		Total
Breastfeeding	n	%	n	%	n	%	N
	372	72.2	127	24.7	16	3.1	515

Source: Fieldwork

Table 37 shows the distribution of time breastfed, 89.4% of adolescents were breastfed for 5-24 months of .

Table 37. Percentage distribution of the time the adolescent was breastfed.

Duration

	N	%
0 - 4 months	25	5.0
5 - 12 months	230	46.2
12 - 24 months	215	43.2
more than 24 months	28	5.6
Total	**498**	**100.0**

Source: Fieldwork

Table 38 shows the distribution of bottle-feeding initiation, 20.3% of bottle-fed adolescents started bottle-feeding at 0 months of age.

Table 38. Percentage distribution of bottle-feeding initiation.

Home

	N	%
0 months	29	20.3
1 month	19	13.3
2 months	6	4.2
3 months	6	4.2
4 months	7	4.9
5 months	8	5.6
6 months	21	14.7
7 months	9	6.3
8 months	15	10.5
9 months	6	4.2
10 months	0	0.0
11 months	1	0.7
12 months	16	11.2
Total	143	100.0
		Source: Fieldwork

Table 39 presents the distribution of exclusive breastfeeding, 80.4% of adolescents were exclusively breastfed for the first six months of life.

Percentage distribution of exclusive breastfeeding during the first six months.

Exclusive breastfeeding

	N	%
Yes	414	80.4
No	101	19.6
Total	515	100.0

Source: Fieldwork

Table 40 shows the distribution of the age at the beginning of the introduction of soft drinks to the diet, 41.4% start drinking soft drinks between 5 and 12 months of age.

Table 40. Percentage distribution of age of initiation of soft drink introduction.

Refreshment

	N	%
0 - 4 months	11	2.2
5 - 12 months	206	41.4
12 - 24 months	194	39.0
more than 24 months	104	20.9
Total	515	103.4

Source: Fieldwork Table 41 shows the distribution of the first foods that were used.

In complementary feeding, 62.1% of adolescents had inadequate complementary feeding.

Table 41. Percentage distribution of the first foods other than milk that were incorporated into the adolescent's diet.

First foods

	N	%
Inadequate	320	62.1
Moderately adequate	124	24.1
Adequate	71	13.8
Total	515	86.2

Source: Fieldwork

Table 42 shows the distribution of body mass index for adolescent age, 27.2% of adolescents were overweight or obese.

Table 42. Percentage distribution of body mass index for age in adolescents.

Body mass index for age

	N	%
Obesity	32	6.2
Overweight	108	21.0
Normal weight	336	65.2
Thinness	35	6.8
Severe thinness	4	0.8
Total	515	100.0

Source: Fieldwork Table 43 shows the distribution of nutritional status according to the In terms of height-for-age indicator for adolescents, 64.1% of adolescents had some degree of low height.

Percentage distribution of height-for-age in adolescents.

Size for age

	N	%
Slightly high	4	0.8
Normal height	181	35.1
Slightly low	221	42.9
Baja	109	21.2
Total	515	100.0

Source: Fieldwork

Table 44 shows the distribution of lower limbs in adolescents, 17.9% of adolescents had short lower limbs (brachyskeletal).

Percentage distribution of lower extremities in adolescents.

Lower extremities

	N	%
Brachyskeletal	92	17.9
Mesoskeletal	164	31.8
Macroskeletal	259	50.3
Total	515	100.0

Source: Fieldwork Table 45 shows the waist-to-height ratio in adolescents, 30.9% of the adolescents were in the same age group as the rest of the population, and 30.9% were in the same age group. adolescents were at high risk of developing chronic degenerative diseases.

Percentage distribution of waist-to-height ratio in adolescents.

Waist index size

	N	%
Acceptable	356	69.1
Elevated	159	30.9
Total	515	100.0

Source: Fieldwork

Table 46 shows a distribution of the adolescent's mother's body mass index, 73.9% of the mothers were overweight or obese.

Table 46. Percentage distribution of body mass index of mothers of adolescents.

Body Mass Index

	N	%
Obesity	109	30.5
Overweight	155	43.4
Adequate	88	24.7
Malnutrition	5	1.4
Total	357	100.0

Source: Fieldwork Table 47 shows the distribution of short limbs of the mother of the adolescent, 50.7% of the mothers had short limbs or also called brachycephalic.

Table 47. Percentage distribution of lower extremities in mothers of adolescents.

Lower extremities

	N	%
Brachyskeletal	174	50.7
Mesoskeletal	109	31.8
Macroskeletal	60	17.5
Total	343	100.0

Source: Fieldwork

Table 48 presents a distribution of the waist-to-height ratio of the mothers of adolescents, 88.3% of the mothers have a high risk of developing chronic degenerative diseases.

Percentage distribution of waist-to-height ratio in mothers of adolescents.

Waist index size

	N	%
Acceptable	42	11.7
Elevated	317	88.3
Total	359	100.0

Source: Fieldwork Table 49 shows a distribution of the body mass index of the father of the 90.2% of parents were overweight or obese.

Table 49. Percentage distribution of body mass index of parents of adolescents.

Body Mass Index

	N	%
Obesity	5	9.8
Overweight	24	47.1
Adequate	22	43.1
Total	51	100.0

Source: Fieldwork

Table 50 shows the distribution of short limbs of the adolescent's father, 31.1% of fathers had short limbs, brachycephalic. **Table 50. Percentage distribution of lower limbs in adolescents.**

Lower extremities

	N	%
Brachyskeletal	14	31.1
Mesoskeletal	15	33.3
Macroskeletal	16	35.6
Total	45	100.0

Source: Fieldwork Table 51 presents a distribution of the waist-to-height ratio of the fathers of the adolescents, 86.3% of fathers are at high risk of developing chronic degenerative diseases.

Table 51. Percentage distribution of waist-height index in parents of adolescents

Waist index size

	N	%
Acceptable	7	13.7
Elevated	44	86.3
Total	51	100.0

Source: Fieldwork

Tables 52 and 53 present the nutritional status according to body mass index for age in pre-school and adolescence, 21.7% of the adolescents showed an unfavourable evolution.

Table 52. Percentage distribution of nutritional status by body mass index for age in preschool and adolescence.

Nutritional status body mass index between age

Nutritional status body mass index by age in adolescence at the stage preschoo servere Obesity Overweight Normal Thinness Thinness

Obesity	4	6	8	1	0	19
Overweight	10	22	49	4	0	85
Normal	16	75	264	26	4	385
Weight	2	4	12	4	0	22
Thinness	0	1	3	0	0	4
Severe thinness						
Total	32	108	336	35	4	515

P=.048

Table 53. Percentage distribution of the evolution of nutritional status according to body mass index for age in pre-school and adolescence.

Evolution n%

Favourable	336	65.2
Intermediate	67	13.0
Unfavourable	112	21.7

Tables 54 and 55 present the nutritional status according to the height-for-age indicator in pre-school and adolescence, 21.2% of adolescents showed an unfavourable evolution.

Table 54. Percentage distribution of nutritional status by height-for-age indicator in preschool and adolescence.

Nutritional status height-for-age at the stage

Nutritional status according to height-for-age in adolescence preschool

Slightly high Normal height Slightly low Total Discharge

Normal	2	46	25	6	79
Slight	2	92	82	14	190
Moderate	0	35	87	57	179
Serious	0	8	27	32	67
Total	4	181	221	108	515

P=.000

Table 55. Percentage distribution of the evolution of nutritional status according to the height-for-age indicator in preschool and adolescence.

Developments n %

Favourable	185	35.9
Intermediate	221	42.9
Unfavourable	109	21.2
Total	515	100.0

Table 56 shows the risk of obesity in adolescence if you have short lower limbs (brachycephalic) and a weekly household income of less than or equal to 500 pesos.

Table 56. Multiple logistic regression model of nutrition status by adolescent BMI-for-age (obesity)
Confidence interval of

B (95%)
Variables Categories Coefficient B (ES) Sig

Inferior				Odds Ratio	Top
Obesity	-0.328 (0.507)	0.520			
Extremities Brachyskeletal	1.332 (0.516)	0.010	1.378	3.789	10.418
lower in Mesoskeletal adolescent Macroskeletal	0.037 (0.537) 0b	0.950 .	0.362 .	1.038	2.973 .
Waist index Acceptable	-3.904 (0.635)	0.000	0.006	0.02	0.07
size of the Elevated	0b	.	.		.
Low weight at Underweight	-0.362 (0.629)	0.570	0.203	0.696	2.387
born of the Normal weight	0b	.	.		.
<= 500 pesos	-1.177 (0.584)	0.040	0.098	0.308	0.967

a. The reference category is: Normal.
b. This parameter is set to zero because it is redundant.

Table 57 presents the risk of becoming overweight in adolescence if you become underweight at birth.

Table 57. Multiple logistic regression model of nutrition status by adolescent BMI-for-age (overweight)

Confidence interval

Coef. B Variables Categories Sig. (ES)	of B (95%) Odds		
	Inferior	Ratio	Top
0.446 (0.345)			
0.665 Brachyskeletal0.060	0.987	1.944	3.828
lower by0.285 Mesoskeletal0.340	0.743	1.33	2.379
Macroskeletal 0b .	.		.
-2.524 Waist to size ratio of Acceptable0.000	0.048	0.08	0.135
teenager Elevated0b .	.		.
-0.905 Low birth weightLow birth weight0.050	0.167	0.405	0.981
of the adolescent Normal weight 0b .	.		.
-0.246 <= 500 pesos 0.480	0.394	0.782	1.551
Family income to the week 0.280	0.354	0.691	1.348
>= 1001 pesos0b .	.		.

a. The reference category is: Normal.

b. This parameter is set to zero because it is redundant.

Table 58 shows that the risk of becoming thin or severely thin in adolescence increases if they have a low birth weight.

Table 58. Multiple logistic regression model of nutritional status by BMI-for-age in adolescents (lean and severely lean)

Confidence Interval of B (95%)

Variables Categories Coefficient B (ES) Sig.

Inferior				Odds Ratio	Top
Thinness and thinness	-3.033 (0.827)	0.000			
severe Extremities Brachyskeletal	-2.101 (1.036)	0.040	0.016	0.122	0.932
lower in Mesoskeletal adolescent Macroskeletal	-1.076 (0.472) 0b	0.020 .	0.135 .	0.341	0.859 .
Waist index Acceptable	1.264 (0.759)	0.100	0.799	3.539	15.665
size of the Elevated	0b	.	.		.
Low weight atUnderweight	1.16 (0.431)	0.010	1.37	3.189	7.422
born of the Normal weight	0b	.	.		.
<= 500 pesos	-0.689 (0.528)	0.190	0.178	0.502	1.414

a. The reference category is: Normal.

b. This parameter is set to zero because it is redundant.

Table 59 shows the risk of mild stunting in adolescence if you develop brachyskeletal or mesoskeletal lower limbs in adolescence and moderate or severe stunting in pre-school.

Table 59. Multiple logistic regression model of adolescent height-for-age nutritional status (slightly low)
Confidence Interval of B (95%)
Variables Categories Coefficient B (ES)Sig.

Inferior				Odds Ratio	Top
Slightly low	0.627 (0.673)	0.352			
Obesity	-1.794 (0.701)	0.010	0.042	0.166	0.657
Mass index Overweight	-0.838 (0.552)	0.129	0.147	0.433	1.277
body for the Normal	-0.357 (0.461)	0.439	0.283	0.7	1.729
age in the					
Adolescent Thinness more					
thinness	0b	.	.		.
severe					
Brachyskeletal	1.072 (0.341)	0.002	1.497	2.922	5.704
lower in Mesoskeletal	0.652 (0.247)	0.008	1.182	1.919	3.116
Adolescent Macroskeletal	0b	.	.		.
Waist index Acceptable	-0.768 (0.331)	0.02	0.243	0.464	0.887
Adolescent High	0b	.	.		.

Confidence interval of B

					(95%)	
Variables	Categories	Coef. B (EN)	Sig.			
			Odds Lower Upper			
					Ratio	
Normal		0b	.	.		.
Size for Mild		0.51 (0.303)	0.092	0.92	1.666	3.017
the age of the Moderate		1.657 (0.337)	0.000	2.706	5.242	10.154
Serious		1.895 (0.492)	0.000	2.536	6.654	17.464
Number of Children <= 2 children		-0.725 (0.464)	0.118	0.195	0.484	1.203
born						
living of the 3 to 7 children		-0.67 (0.353)	0.057	0.256	0.512	1.021
mother of the						
adolescent>= 8 children		0b	.	.		.

a. The reference category is: Normal.

b. This parameter is set to zero because it is redundant.

Table 60 shows the risk of low height in adolescence if brachycephalic lower limbs and moderate and severe height-for-age in pre-school.

Table 60. Multiple logistic regression model of adolescent height-for-age nutritional status (low)

Confidence Interval of B (95%)

Variables Categories Coefficient B (ES) Sig

Inferior				Odds Ratio	Top
Baja	0.784 (0.864)	0.364			
Obesity	-3.242 (0.862)	0	0.007	0.039	0.212
Mass index Overweight	-2.473 (0.699)	0	0.021	0.084	0.332
body for the Normal age in the adolescent Thinness more	-0.976 (0.543)	0.072	0.13	0.377	1.092
thinness	0b	.	.		.
severe					
Extremities Brachyskeletal	1.864 (0.415)	0	2.861	6.452	14.547
lower in Mesoskeletal	0.257 (0.357)	0.471	0.643	1.293	2.602
Adolescent Macroskeletal	0b	.	.		.
Waist index Acceptable	-2.296 (0.413)	0	0.045	0.101	0.226
size of the					
Adolescent High	0b	.	.		.

Continue...

Confidence interval of B (95%)

Variables Categories Coefficient B (ES) Sig

Inferior					Odds Ratio	Top
	Normal	0b	.	.		.
Size for	Slight	0.147 (0.55)	0.789	0.394	1.158	3.402
the age of the preschool	Moderate	2.714 (0.522)	0	5.418	15.085	41.998
	Serious	3.572 (0.635)	0	10.259	35.586	123.434
Number of	<= 2 children	-0.734 (0.636)	0.248	0.138	0.48	1.668
children born	3 to 7 children	-0.563 (0.438)	0.199	0.241	0.57	1.344
living in the						
mother of the	>= 8 children	0b	.	.		.

a. The reference category is: Normal.

b. This parameter is set to zero because it is redundant.

CHAPTER 4

DISCUSSION

The population studied has 30.3% more children under five years of age with short stature compared to the prevalence reported by the ENSANUT 2018-19 for rural communities, which tells us that these communities in the Mazahua zone have poor health, nutrition and living conditions. With regard to the prevalence of overweight and obesity in adolescents, according to the ENSANUT 2018-19, there is a minor difference of 11.2%, since, according to the survey, 38.4% of the national population has these conditions, while 27.2% of the population studied had these conditions. The associations that were significant were: short stature at preschool age is associated with short stature at adolescent age, as well as short lower limbs at adolescent age. The acceptable waist-to-height ratio at adolescent age was found to be a protective factor against overweight and obesity at the same age. In relation to socio-economic conditions, three of them showed an association with adolescent nutritional status: live births, low weight and weekly family income.

CONCLUSIONS

Childhood nutritional status has a stronger association with possible effects on height at adolescent age than BMI/e.Short stature and short limbs are associated with overweight and obesity adolescence. While having an acceptable waist-to-height ratio decreases the likelihood of being overweight and obese.It is necessary to study the current diet of adolescents in order to know the effect it has on their nutritional status at that age; food insecurity and/or the obesogenic environment play an important role in this condition. In addition, pre-post-natal and socio-economic data should be studied at pre-school age; it should be noted that 72% of the families participating in this study are concentrated in the marginal and lower categories according to socio-economic level.Many of the families interviewed are in poor socio-economic conditions, such as overcrowding (31.2%), use of firewood for cooking (86.8%), open fire or oven without chimney or hood (39.0%), the toilets they use cannot be flushed (59.6%), they have no rubbish collection service so they choose to burn it (67.6%), they have no social security (89.6%), etcetera. It is necessary to carry out timely nutritional surveillance, which should have the capacity to collect more specific information in real time, allowing for a better understanding of the conditions in which children develop and the possibility of intervening in the health and poverty cycle instantaneously. Decent, decentralised and strategically distributed health systems in the most unprotected territories are a necessity in the face of the evident public health problems in the country. It is vitally important to create public policies that guarantee maternal and perinatal health, family planning, and improve the income of families in the country's rural communities, as well as their social conditions in order to reduce stunting in preschool age, overweight and obesity in adolescence, and chronic non-degenerative diseases in adulthood.

REFERENCES BIBLIOGRAPHIC

Chávez & Muñoz. (2007). Malnutrition "its impact on human health and functional capacity" (Universidad Autónoma del Estado de Morelos., Ed.; Primera).

Cravioto (2003). Desnutrición Infantil en México. Fundación Derechos de La Infancia.

Cuevas-Nasu, L., García-Guerra, A., González-Castell, L. D., Morales-Ruan, M. del C., Humarán, I. M. G., Gaona-Pineda, E. B., García-Feregrino, R., Rodríguez-Ramírez, S., Gómez-Acosta, L. M., Ávila-Arcos, M. A., Shamah-Levy, T., & Rivera-Dommarco, J. (2021). Magnitude and trend of undernutrition and factors associated with low height in children under five in Mexico, Ensanut 2018-19. Salud Publica de Mexico, 63(3), 339-349. https://doi.org/10.21149/12193

Frongillo, E. A., Leroy, J. L., & Lapping, K. (2019). Appropriate Use of Linear Growth Measures to Assess Impact of Interventions on Child Development and Catch-Up Growth. In Advances in Nutrition (Vol. 10, Issue 3, pp. 372-379). Oxford University Press. https://doi.org/10.1093/advances/nmy093

Garibay-Nieto & Miranda-Lora. (2008). Impact of fetal programming and nutrition during the first year of life on the development of obesity and its complications (Vol. 65). www.medigraphic.com

Labraña, A. M., Ramírez-Alarcón, K., Troncoso-Pantoja, C., Leiva, A. M., Villagrán, M., Mardones, L., Lasserre-Laso, N., Martorell, M., Lanuza-Rilling, F., Petermann-Rocha, F., Martínez-Sanguinetti, M. A., & Celis-Morales, C. (2020). Childhood obesity: The benefits of breastfeeding versus formula feeding. In Revista Chilenade Nutricion (Vol. 47, Issue 3, pp. 478-483). Sociedad Chilena de Nutricion Bromatologia y Toxilogica. https://doi.org/10.4067/S0717-75182020000300478

Leroy, J. L., Ruel, M., & Habicht, J. P. (2013). Critical windows for nutritional interventions against stunting. In American Journal of Clinical Nutrition (Vol. 98, Issue 3, pp. 854-855). https://doi.org/10.3945/ajcn.113.066647

Malina R. M., Peña Reyes M. E., Swee Kheng Tan, Buschang P. H., Little B. B., & Koziel S. (2004). Secular change in height, sitting height and leg length in rural Oaxaca,southern Mexico: 1968-2000 (Vol. 31). www.tandf.co.uk

Monteiro, P. O. A., Victora, C. G., Barros, F. C., & Monteiro, L. M. A. (2003). Birth size, early childhood growth, and adolescent obesity in a Brazilian birth cohort. International Journal of Obesity, 27(10), 1274-1282. https://doi.org/10.1038/sj.ijo.0802409

Moreno-Villares, J. M., & Dalmau, J. (2001). Alterations in foetal nutrition and long-term effects: more than a hypothesis? https://www.researchgate.net/publication/242666452

Prentice, A. M., Ward, K. A., Goldberg, G. R., Jarjou, L. M., Moore, S. E., Fulford, A. J., & Prentice, A. (2013). Critical windows for nutritional interventions against stunting. In American Journal of Clinical Nutrition (Vol. 97, Issue 5, pp. 911-918). https://doi.org/10.3945/ajcn.112.052332

Ravasco, P., Anderson, H., Mardones, F., & Ravasco, P. (2010). Methods for assessing nutritional status. Nutr Hosp Supl, 3(3), 57-66.

Shamah. (2018). National Health and Nutrition Survey, National Results.
Shamah & Rivera (2020). National Health and Nutrition Survey 2020 on Covid-19 National Results.
UNICEF. (2019). THE CHILDREN'S AND ADOLESCENTS' AGENDA.ùwww.unicef.org/mexico/media/306/file/agenda%20de%20la%20infancia%20 https://y%20la%20adolescencia%202019-2024.pdf
Wagstaff, A. (2002). Policy and Practice Theme Papers Poverty and health sector inequalities *. Bolletin of the World Health Organization, 97-105. www.cmhealth.org/wg1_paper5.pdf

ANNEXES

Information gathering instrument

UNICLA UNIVERSIDAD CONTEMPORÁNEA DE LAS AMÉRICAS

Asociación entre el estado de nutrición en preescolares y la adolescencia en localidades rurales del Estado de México, 2002 - 2022.

1.– DATOS DE IDENTIFICACIÓN

1.1 Número de encuesta:__________

1.2 Nombre del municipio:______________________________

1.3 Clave INEGI municipio:__________

1.4 Nombre de la localidad:______________________________

1.5 Clave INEGI localidad:__________

1.6 Fecha de visita:______________________________
Día / Mes / Año

1.7 Clave ID SCPIAN: __________

2.- IDENTIFICACIÓN DEL ADOLESCENTE

2.1 Nombre del entrevistado:______________________________
NOMBRE(S) APELLIDO PATERNO APELLIDO MATERNO

2.2 Nombre del adolescente:______________________________
NOMBRE(S) APELLIDO PATERNO APELLIDO MATERNO

2.3 CURP:______________________________

2.4 Fecha de nacimiento: ______________
Día / Mes / Año

2.5 Sexo: **M** **F** Marco con una X, **M** si es masculino **F** si es femenino

3.– CARACTERÍSTICAS DE LA VIVIENDA

1.- ¿De qué material es la mayor parte del techo de su vivienda?, solo un código.

1.- Material de desecho
2.- Lámina de cartón
3.- Lámina metálica
4.- Lámina de asbesto
5.- Palma o paja
6.- Madera o tejamanil
7.- Terrado con viguería
8.- Teja
9.- Losa de concreto o viguetas con bovedilla

2.- ¿De qué material es la mayor parte de las paredes o muros de su vivienda?, solo un código.

1.- Material de desecho
2.- Lámina de cartón
3.- Lámina de asbesto o metálica
4.- Carrizo, bambú o palma
5.- Embarro, bajareque o paja
6.- Madera
7.- Adobe
8.- Tabique, ladrillo, *block*, piedra, cantera, cemento o concreto

3.- ¿De qué material es la mayor parte del piso de su vivienda?

1.– Tierra
2.– Cemento o firme
3.- Madera, mosaico u otro

4.- **¿Cuántos cuartos se usan para dormir sin contar pasillos ni baños?**

1.- Anote el número

5.- En total, ¿cuántos cuartos tiene esta vivienda (no cuente pasillos ni baños)?

1.- Anote el número

6.- ¿Cuántas personas duermen habitualmente en la vivienda?

1.- Anote el número

9.– ¿En el cuarto donde cocinan, también duermen?

(1=SÍ, 2=NO)

7.– Observar o preguntar si en la vivienda hay: (1=SÍ, 2=NO)

(admite más de una respuesta)

1.– Ventilación
2.– Animales adentro
3.– Energía eléctrica
4.– Cocina separada

(Si en la opción 4 la respuesta es 2 pase a la pregunta 9, si la respuesta es 1 pase a la pregunta 8)

8.– Entonces, ¿cocinan los alimentos... (Leer y selecciona un solo rectángulo)

1.– en un pasillo o corredor?
2.– en un tejaban o techito?
3.– al aire libre?
} Pasa a la 10

4.– ¿No cocinan en esta vivienda? Pasa a la 12

Continuar...

10.- ¿El combustible que más usan para cocinar es…

Lee y cruza un código

1.– leña? ☐
2.– carbón? ☐
3.- gas de cilindro o estacionario? ☐
4.- gas natural o de tubería? ☐
5.– electricidad? ☐
6.- ¿Otro combustible? ☐
7.- ¿No cocinan? ☐ Pasa a la 12

11.- ¿Qué tipo de estufa utilizan para cocinar o calentar alimentos? Lee y cruza un código

1.– Estufa o parrilla de gas ☐
2.– Estufa o parrilla eléctrica ☐
3.- Fuego abierto u horno sin chimenea ni campana ☐
4.- Fuego abierto u horno con chimenea o campana ☐
5.– Horno cerrado con chimenea ☐
6.- Otro (especifica) ☐
7.- ____________________

12.– ¿Esta vivienda tiene agua entubada… (Leer y selecciona un solo rectángulo)

1.– dentro de la vivienda? ☐
2.– solo en el terreno? ☐
3.– ¿No tiene agua entubada? ☐ Pasa a la 14

13.– ¿El agua entubada que llega a su vivienda viene… (Leer y selecciona un solo rectángulo)

1.– del servicio público de agua? ☐
2.– de un pozo? ☐
3.– de una pipa? ☐
4.– de otra vivienda? ☐
5.– de otro lugar? ☐
6.– ____________________ Especifica

Pasa a la 15

14.– Entonces, ¿el agua que usan en esta vivienda...(Leer y selecciona un solo rectángulo)

1.– la sacan o acarrean de un pozo? ☐
2.– la acarrean de una toma o llave comunitaria? ☐
3.– la traen de otra vivienda? ☐
4.– la trae una pipa? ☐
5.– la acarrean de un río, arroyo o lago? ☐
6.– la captan de la lluvia? ☐

15.– ¿Cómo es la disposición de excretas en la vivienda? (Leer y selecciona un solo rectángulo)

1.– Drenaje de la red pública ☐
2.– Fosa séptica o tanque séptico (biodigestor) ☐
3.– Tubería que va a dar a una barranca o grieta ☐
4.– Tubería que va a dar a un río, lago o mar? ☐
5.– Fecalismo a ras de suelo ☐

16.– **¿Cuántos baños tiene esta vivienda con excusado y regadera?**

1.- Anote el número ☐☐

18.– ¿Este servicio sanitario lo comparten con otra vivienda?

Cruza un código

1.– Sí ☐
2.– No ☐

17.– ¿El servicio sanitario...

Lee y cruza un código

1.– tiene descarga directa de agua? ☐
2.– le echan agua con cubeta? ☐
3.– no se le puede echar agua? ☐

19.– ¿La basura de esta vivienda...

(Leer y selecciona la opción más frecuente)

1.– la recoge un camión o carrito de basura? ☐
2.– la tiran en el basurero público? ☐
3.– la tiran en un contenedor o depósito? ☐
4.– la queman? ☐
5.– La entierran? ☐
6.– la tiran en un terreno baldío o calle? ☐
7.– la tiran a la barranca o grieta? ☐
8.– la tiran al río, lago o presa? ☐

20.– ¿Esta vivienda...

Lee y cruza un código

1.– es rentada? ☐
2.– es prestada? ☐
3.– es propia pero la están pagando? ☐
4.– es propia? ☐
5.– está intestada o en litigio? ☐
6.– está en otra situación? ☐

21.– **¿Esta hogar cuenta con…**

(1=SI, 2=NO)

1.– **Internet?** ☐
2.– **automóvil?** ☐
3.– **camioneta cerrada o con cabina?** ☐
4.– **camioneta de caja?** ☐

4.– RECURSOS PARA LA ALIMENTACIÓN FAMILIAR

1.- ¿Cuánto es el ingreso económico familiar a la semana?

$____________________

2.- ¿Cuánto gasta la familia a la semana en alimentos?

$____________________

3.– ¿La familia, o alguno de sus miembros reciben algún tipo de ayuda alimentaria en el ultimo mes?

Cruza un código

1.– Sí ☐
2.– No ☐ Pasa a la 5

4.- ¿Cuáles?

1.– Despensas del DIF ☐
2.– Despensas de alguna ONG ☐
3.– Desayunos escolares fríos ☐
4.– Desayunos escolares calientes ☐
5.– Comedor comunitario ☐
6.- Leche LICONSA ☐
7.– Otro ____________________ Especifica

Continuar...

5.– ¿A lo largo de la vida de (nombre del adolescente) recibió algún tipo de ayuda alimentaria?

Cruza un código 1.– Sí ☐ 2.– No ☐ Pasa a la 7

6.- ¿Cuál?

1.– Despensas del DIF ☐
2.– Despensas de alguna ONG ☐
3.– Desayunos escolares fríos ☐
4.– Desayunos escolares calientes ☐
5.– Comedor comunitario ☐
6.- Leche LICONSA ☐
7.– Oportunidades ☐
8.– Prospera ☐
9.– Progresa ☐
10.– Otro ________ Especifica

7.– ¿Cría animales para la alimentación?

Cruza un código 1.– Sí ☐ 2.– No ☐ Pasa a la 8

7.2.- ¿De que tipo?	7.3.– Autoconsumo	7.4.– Venta	7.5.– Ambos
1.– Ganado menor	☐	☐	☐
2.– Ganado mayor	☐	☐	☐
3.– Otro________	☐	☐	☐

8.– ¿Cultiva alimentos?

Cruza un código 1.– Sí ☐ 2.– No ☐ Pasa a la sección 5

8.2.- ¿De que tipo?	8.3.– Autoconsumo	8.4.– Venta	8.5.– Ambos
1.– Frutales	☐	☐	☐
2.– Hortalizas	☐	☐	☐
3.– Granos básicos	☐	☐	☐

5.– DATOS GENERALES DE LOS PADRES Y ADOLESCENTE

1.- Mamá del adolescente

1. Edad:________ (Años cumplidos) 2. Número de hijos:_____ (Nacidos vivos) 3. Estado Civil:______________ 4. Idioma:________________ (1= Indígena, 2= Español, 3= Bilingüe)

5. Seguridad Social:_____________ (¿Cómo se llama?) 6. **¿Hasta qué año o grado aprobó (NOMBRE) en la escuela?**:_______ (Terminada)

2. Papá del adolescente

1. Edad:__________ (Años cumplidos) 2. Estado Civil:_______ 3. Idioma:___________ (1= Indígena, 2= Español, 3= Bilingüe) 4. Seguridad Social:_______________ (¿Cómo se llama?)

5. **¿Hasta qué año o grado aprobó (NOMBRE) en la escuela?**:_______________ (Terminada)

3.- Adolescente

1. Edad:___________ (Años cumplidos) 2. Número de hijos:_____ (Nacidos vivos) 3. Estado Civil:______________ 4. Idioma:_______________ (1= Indígena, 2= Español, 3= Bilingüe)

5. Seguridad Social:_____________ (¿Cómo se llama?) 6. ¿Estado fisiológico?:_______ (1. Embarazada, 2 Dando pecho y 3. Ambos)

7. **¿Hasta qué año o grado aprobó (NOMBRE) en la escuela?**:_______________

8. **¿Quién es el jefe de familia en el hogar?**: Papá _____ o Mamá ___ (Marca con una **X**)

9. **De todas las personas de más de 14 años que viven en el hogar, ¿cuántas trabajaron en el último mes?**:________

6.– INFORMACIÓN POSTNATAL DEL ADOLESCENTE

1. El adolescente tuvo un tiempo de gestación:________ Meses 2. Peso al nacer:____________ (Kg)

1.– **Normal** 38 a 42 semanas, 2.– **Prematuro** menos de 37 semanas y 3.– **Posmaduro** más de 42 semanas.

3.– ¿Fue alimentado al seno materno? Cruza un código 1.– Sí ☐ 2.– No ☐

4. ¿Durante cuantos meses?:_____

5.– ¿Fue alimentado regularmente con leche en biberón los primeros 12 meses? Cruza un código 1.– Sí ☐ 2.– No ☐

6. Si la respuesta anterior fue SI ¿A que edad inicio?:_____ Meses

7. ¿A que edad recibió por primera vez otro alimento distinto a la leche materna?:_____ Meses

8.– ¿Durante los primeros 6 meses de vida sólo fue alimentado al seno materno? Cruza un código 1.– Sí ☐ 2.– No ☐

Continuar...

9. ¿Cuáles son los alimentos solidos con que inicio la alimentación complementaria?:____________________
(Por lo menos menciona tres alimentos)

10. ¿A qué edad probo el refresco por primera vez?:________________ Meses

7.– ANTROPOMETRÍA

1 Adolescente

1 Peso:____________ Kilogramos 2 Talla:____________ Centímetros 3 Talla sentado:____________ Centímetros

4 Circunferencia de cintura:____________ Centímetros

2 Mamá del adolescente

1 Peso:____________ Kilogramos 2 Talla:____________ Centímetros 3 Talla sentado:____________ Centímetros

4 Circunferencia de cintura:____________ Centímetros

3 Papá del adolescente

1 Peso:____________ Kilogramos 2 Talla:____________ Centímetros 3 Talla sentado:____________ Centímetros

4 Circunferencia de cintura:____________ Centímetros

CONFIDENCIALIDAD

Conforme a las disposiciones del **Artículo 37, párrafo primero de la Ley del Sistema Nacional de Información Estadística y Geográfica** en vigor: "Los datos que proporcionen para fines estadísticos los Informantes del Sistema a las Unidades en términos de la presente Ley, serán estrictamente confidenciales y bajo ninguna circunstancia podrán utilizarse para otro fin que no sea el estadístico."

OBLIGATORIEDAD

De acuerdo con el **Artículo 45, párrafo primero, de la Ley del Sistema Nacional de Información Estadística y Geográfica** en vigor: "Los informantes del Sistema estarán obligados a proporcionar, con veracidad y oportunidad, los datos e informes que les soliciten las autoridades competentes para fines estadísticos, censales y geográficos, y prestarán apoyo a las mismas".

RESPETO A LAS PERSONAS

De acuerdo al Artículo 13, párrafo primero del Reglamento de la Ley General de Salud en materia de Investigación para la Salud, en vigor; "En toda investigación en la que el ser humano sea sujeto de estudio, deberán prevalecer el criterio del respeto a su dignidad y la protección a sus derechos y bienestar".

Letter of informed settlement

UNICLA

CARTA DE ASENTIMIENTO INFORMADO

Asociación entre el estado de nutrición en preescolares y la adolescencia en localidades rurales del Estado de México, 2002 - 2022

El objetivo general: "Evaluar el estado de nutrición en la edad adolescente y compararlo con el estado de nutrición que presentaban en edad preescolar en población de localidades rurales del Estado de México".

Para llevar a cabo los objetivos del estudio es necesario que nos permitas realizar los siguientes procedimientos:

1. La aplicación de una encuesta que está dividida en los siguientes apartados: datos de identificación, identificación del adolescente, características de la vivienda, recursos para la alimentación familiar, datos generales de los padres y adolescentes, Información postnatal del adolescente y antropometría.
2. La toma de peso, talla, talla sentado y circunferencia de cintura del adolescente, así como del papá y mamá del adolescente.

Hola mi nombre es ______________________________ y estudio o colaboro en la Universidad Contemporánea de las Américas en el doctorado en Salud Pública. Actualmente se está realizando un estudio para conocer acerca de **la asociación entre el estado de nutrición en preescolares y la adolescencia,** y para ello queremos pedirte que nos apoyes.

Tu participación en el estudio consistiría en responder una encuesta con ayuda de tu tutor o responsable, así como la toma de medidas de peso, talla, talla sentado y circunferencia de cintura.

Tu participación en el estudio es voluntaria, es decir, aun cuando tus papá o mamá hayan dicho que puedes participar, si tú no quieres hacerlo puedes decir que no. Es tu decisión si participas o no en el estudio. También es importante que sepas que, si en un momento dado ya no quieres continuar en el estudio, no habrá ningún problema, o si no quieres responder a alguna pregunta en particular, tampoco habrá problema.

Toda la información que nos proporciones/ las mediciones que realicemos nos ayudarán a conocer si existe una asociación entre el estado de nutrición en preescolares y la adolescencia.

Esta información será confidencial. Esto quiere decir que no diremos a nadie tus respuestas (O RESULTADOS DE MEDICIONES), sólo lo sabrán las personas que forman parte del equipo de este estudio y tus padres.

Operationalisation of variables

Variable	Type of variable	Conceptual definition	Dimensions	Indicators
State from	Depende nt	Through the indicators	1.- Size 2.- Weight	1.- BMI 2.- BMI/E
nutrition		anthropometri	3.-	3.- Waist
anthropome		mass index	waist	size
of the adolescent		body mass index for age	4.- Seated size	4.- I.E.
		it is possible		
		diagnose the		
		nutritional		
		if you are		
		normal weight,		
		overweight or		
		obesity.		
		Size indicator		
		age (T/E) if		
		has short		
		normal or high		
		for their age.		
		Waist index		
		risk indicator		
		cardiovascular		
		adolescents,		
		categorise		
		acceptable or		
		high. Index		
		skeletal or		
		Manouvrier		
		relates the		
		of the trunk		
		length of the		
		lower limb,		
		This is		
		the difference		
		height and		
		sitting. The		
		of individuals		
		according to		
		skeletal is:		
		Baraquischelic		
		Mesoskeletal		
		Macroskeletal.		

Variable	Type of variable	Conceptual definition	Dimensions	Indicators
State from Nutrition by anthropometry in at preschool stage	Independent	Via anthropometric indicators Body Mass Index for Age (BMI/Age) it is possible to diagnose the nutritional whether you are underweight, normal weight, overweight, overweight u obesity; and via on height-for-age (T/A) indicator if you are short, normal height or tall for your age.	1.- Size 2.- Weight 3.- Age	1.- Size for age 2.- Weight for age
Socio-economic index	Independent	It is the set of economic, sociological, educational and occupational variables by which an individual or group is and labour variables by which an individual or group is classified a social hierarchy.	Socio-economic level of the AMAI 2022, according to 6 variableswhich Integrate the model	1.- Discharge 2.- Medium High 3.- Media 4.- Medium Low 5.- Upper Low 6.- Lower Lower 7.- Marginal

Variable	Type of variable	Conceptual definition	Dimensions	Indicators
Weight at adolescent birth weight	Independent	Birth weight is the weight taken immediately after birth. after birth A low birth birth weight is considered to be one that weighs less than 2.5 kg and a high weight is when it is more than 4 kg.	1.-< 2.500 Kg 2.-=> 2.500 Kg 3.- Don't know or don't remember	1.- Low birth weight 2.- Normal 3.- Don't know or don't remember
Size from parents	Independent	The size represents the sum of the length of the segments and sub-segments of the body, can be used as a reference point when at analyse the proportionality of the body.	1.- Size 2.- Seated size	1.- Total size 2.-Lower extremities
Age from parents	Independent	Time that a person or other being has lived a person or other livingù living being counting from birth	1.- Age in years completed	1.- <30 2.- 30-39 3.- 40-49 4.- >50

Variable	Type of variable	Conceptual definition	Dimensions	Indicators
Marital status of parents	Independent	Marital status is defined the particular condition that Characterises a person in terms of his or her personal links with individuals of the other sex or of the same sex, with whom he or she Will create ties that will be legally recognised even if the same person is not is a relativeo direct relative.	1.- Single 2.- Married 3.- Divorced 4.- Free union 5.- Widower	1.- With a partner 2.- Without a partner
Adolescent's marital status	Independent	Marital status is defined the particular condition that Characterises a person in terms of his or her personal links with individuals of the other sex or of the same sex, with whom he or she will create ties that will be legally recognised even if the same person is not is a relativeor immediate family member.	1.- Single 2.- Married 3.- Divorced 4.- Free union 5.- Widower	1.- With a partner 2.- Without a partner

Variable	Type of variable	Conceptual definition	Dimensions	Indicators
Schooling of parents	Independent	Period of time a person attends school to study and learn, especially the time spent in and learn, especially the time spent in compulsory education. compulsory education.	1.- Illiterate 2.- Can read and write 3.- Incomplete primary education 4.- Complete primary education 5.- Secondary school completed 6.- Completed baccalaureate or equivalent 7.- Technical career 8.- Professional studies	1.- No education 2.- Pre-school 3.- Incomplete primary education 4.- Complete primary education 5.- Incomplete secondary school 6.- Secondary school completed 7.- Incomplete high school 8.- High school completed 9.- Incomplete bachelor's degree 10.- Completed Bachelor's degree 11.- Postgraduate
Schooling of the adolescent	Independent	Period of time a person attends school to study and learn, especially the time spent in and learn, especially the time spent in compulsory education. compulsory education.	1.- Illiterate 2.- Can read and write 3.- Incomplete primary education 4.- Complete primary education 5.- Secondary school completed 6.- Completed baccalaureate or equivalent 7.- Technical career 8.- Professional studies	1.- Illiterate 2.- Alphabet 3.- Basic 4.- Media 5.- Higher or more

Variable	Type of variable	Conceptual definition	Dimensions	Indicators
Social Security	Independent	The protection that a society provides to the individuals and the	1.- IMSS 2.- ISSSTE 3.- PEMEX 4.- SEDENA	1.- IMSS - ISSSTE 2.- Other 3.- No security
		households for	5.- SEMAR	
		ensure the	6.- Private	
		access to the	Insurance	
		medical assistance	Other Institution	
		and security of	8.- No	
		income	Security 9.- Don't Know	
Number of children	Independent	The number of live births	Number of live births	1.- Only Child 2.- Two children 3.- more than or equal to three children
Languag e	Independent	It is a system of	1.- English	1.- Indigenous
		communicatio n	2.- Mazahua	2.- English
		verbal or gestural, characteristic of a human society	3.- Another local language	3.- Bilingual

Dr. Marco Antonio Quiroz Aguilar

Degree in Nutrition from the Universidad Autónoma Metropolitana, Master's degree in Nutrition, Health and Dietetics from the Universidad Autónoma del Estado de Morelos and PhD in Public Health from UNICLA. He is currently researcher A at the Instituto Nacional de Ciencias Médicas y Nutrición Salvador Zubirán and professor at the Universidad Autónoma de Guerrero campus Zona Norte.

Dr. Fernando Axiel Rodríguez Filio

Graduate in Nutrition, Master in Nutrition, Health and Dietetics with specialisation in Community and Social Development and Doctor in Public Health. He was coordinator of Integral Nutrition Programmes in the states of Guerrero, Chiapas and Oaxaca. He coordinated projects and some state and national surveys. He was a teacher-researcher and coordinator of the degree in nutrition in Guerrero. He is currently operational director of the consultancy Nutriendo ConCiencia.

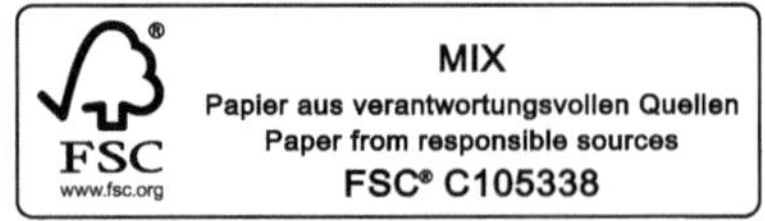

Printed by Books on Demand GmbH, Norderstedt / Germany